The Fruity living Made Easy

Copyright Notice.

Table of contents

Introduction

Welcome to "The Fruity Living"!

Why fruits are Fundamental for maintaining a healthy Life

In today's fast-paced world, it's simple to get caught up within the hustle and bustle and disregard to organize our wellbeing. We are always besieged with handled nourishments, sugary snacks, and fast fixes that guarantee comfort but offer small or no dietary esteem to the body. But what on the off chance that I told you there's a way to alter your wellbeing, boost your vitality, and supercharge your prosperity all through the control of natural products?

The Significance of Normal Nourishment Utilization

Natural products like fruits are more than fair, a delicious nibble or a sound propensity, it's a key to opening our full potential. By joining normal nourishments like fruits into our diets, we're giving our bodies the devices they ought to flourish and stay healthy. We're talking dynamic vitality, gleaming skin, and a resistant framework that's terminating on all barrels. And the leading portion? Fruits are open, reasonable, and tasty!

Grasping a Productive Way of life

Within the pages, we'll take a trip through the brilliant world of fruits, investigating the astonishing benefits of 20 extraordinary fruits and how they can change your life for good. From the antioxidant powerhouse of berries to the tropical euphoria of pineapple, we'll plunge into the dietary profiles, health benefits, and creative ways to appreciate each fruit. Whether you are a natural product aficionado or fair beginning out, this book is your direct way of grasping a productive way of life that will take off you feeling nourished, motivated, and prepared to require the world!

So, are you prepared to connect the productive transformation? Let's plunge in and find the mind blowing world of fruits together!

Apple

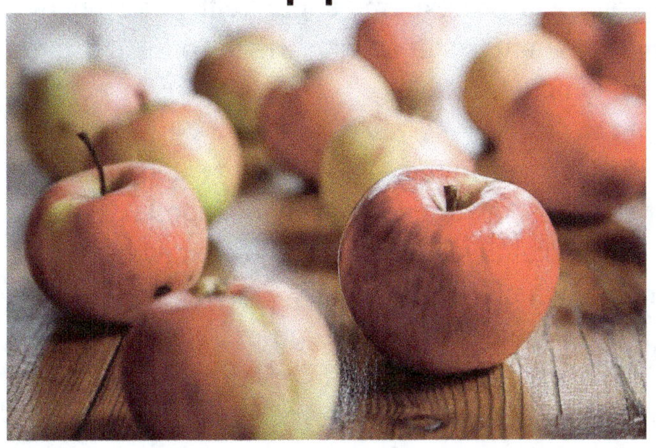

Apple: The Ultimate Super fruit

Dietary Profile: The Lowdown

Meet Apple, the extreme super fruit! This crunchy, juicy enchant is stuffed with a noteworthy cluster of supplements, counting:

-        Fiber: 4 grams per medium sized apple (that's 17% of your day by day dosage!)
-        Vitamin C: 10% of your everyday needs per medium apple
-        Cancer prevention agents: Quercetin, Catechins, and Chromogenic Corrosive (say that three times quick!)
-        Potassium: 5% of your day by day needs per medium apple

Health Benefits: The Great Stuff

- So, what does this supplement powerhouse do for you? Apple's noteworthy resume incorporates:
- Heart Wellbeing: Fiber and cancer prevention agents group up to lower cholesterol and blood weight, keeping your heart upbeat and solid!
- Stomach related Enchant: Fiber makes difference control bowel developments,

avoiding obstruction and keeping your intestine upbeat!
-   Anti-Inflammatory Genius: Quercetin and other cancer prevention agents decrease irritation, facilitating indications of joint pain, sensitivities, and indeed asthma!
-   Brain Control: Apple's cancer prevention agents and fiber back cognitive work, keeping your intellect sharp and centered!

Creative Ways to enjoy: Get Your Apple On!

Prepared to induce your apple on? Attempt these imaginative ways to appreciate:

-   Apple Pie Cereal: Include diced apples to your cereal for a sweet and fulfilling breakfast!
-   Apple Cider Vinegar Tonic: Blend 1 tablespoon of apple cider vinegar with water for a reviving stomach related help!
-   Apple and Brie Flame broiled Cheese: Layer cut apples and brie cheese for a gourmet turn on the classic flame broiled cheese!
-   Apple and Berry Smoothie: Mix apples, solidified berries, and a sprinkle of almond drain for a sound and delicious smoothie!

There you've got it Apple, the extreme super fruit! Whether you appreciate it as a nibble, include it to your top pick formulas, or utilize it as a common cure, Apple is beyond any doubt to bring a burst of enhance and nourishment to your life!

Banana

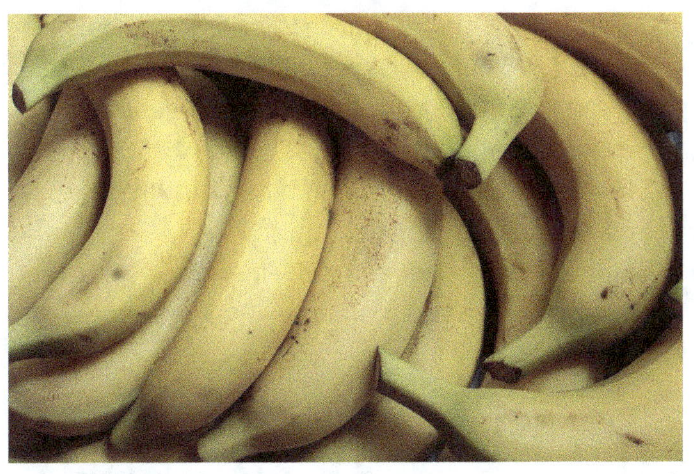

Banana: The Sunshine Fruit

Dietary Profile: The Scoop

Meet Banana, the daylight fruit that's bursting with vitality and goodness! This awe-inspiring, yellow enchant is packed with:

- Potassium: 422 milligrams per medium banana (that's 12% of your everyday dosage!)
- Vitamin C: 10% of your everyday needs per medium banana
- Fiber: 3 grams per medium banana (that's 10% of your day by day dosage!)
- Cancer prevention agents: Phenolic compounds and carotenoids (say that three times quick!)

Health Benefits: The Great Stuff

So, what does this sunny whiz do for you? Banana's amazing resume incorporates:

- Vitality Boost: Potassium and vitamins offer assistance control liquid adjust, keeping your vitality levels taking off!
- Disposition Lifter: Tryptophan and vitamin B6 bolster serotonin generation, making a difference to ease push sand uneasiness!

- Stomach related Charm: Fiber makes a difference direct bowel developments, avoiding obstruction and keeping your intestine upbeat!
- Heart Wellbeing: Potassium and fiber group up to lower blood weight and cholesterol, keeping your heart cheerful and solid!

Creative Ways to enjoy: Go Bananas!

Prepared to go bananas? Attempt these inventive ways to appreciate:

- Banana "Decent" Cream: Solidify bananas and mix into a rich, dairy-free ice cream!
- Banana Oat Hotcakes: Pound ready bananas and blend with oats, eggs, and nectar for a delightful breakfast treat!
- Banana and Shelled Nut Butter Smoothie: Mix bananas, shelled nut butter, and almond drain for a velvety and fulfilling smoothie!
- Banana Chips: Cut bananas lean and heat until fresh for a top notch nibble!

There you've got it; Banana, the daylight fruit that's beyond any doubt to brighten up your day!
Whether you appreciate it as a nibble, include it to your top choice formulas, or utilize it as a

characteristic cure, Bananas are beyond any doubt to bring a burst of vitality and bliss to your life!

Mango

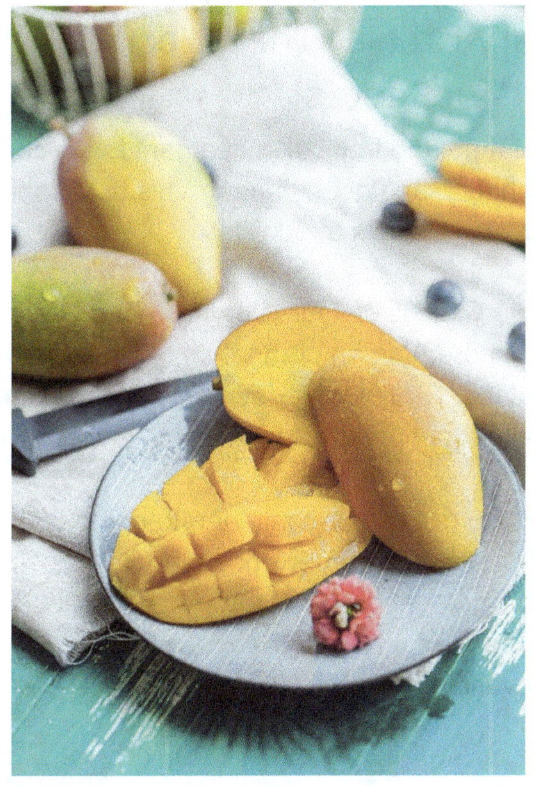

Mango: The Tropical Temptation

Dietary Profile: The Succulent Points of interest

Meet Mango, the tropical enticement that's bursting with enhance and nourishment! This delectable, brilliant enchant is stuffed with:

- Vitamin C: 45% of your everyday needs per glass (that's more than an orange!)
- Vitamin A: 10% of your day by day needs per container (supporting sound vision and resistant work)
- Fiber: 2.6 grams per container (keeping your stomach related framework cheerful and solid) - Cancer prevention agents: Different polyphenols and flavonoids (battling free radicals and aggravation)

Health Benefits: The Sweet Stuff

So, what does this tropical genius do for you? Mango's noteworthy resume incorporates:

- Eye Wellbeing: Vitamin A and cancer prevention agents back sound vision and diminish the hazard of age-related macular degeneration! –

Safe Framework Boost: Vitamin C and cancer prevention agents offer assistance battle off contaminations and keep your safe framework solid!

- Stomach related Charm: Fiber and cancer prevention agents bolster sound absorption, avoiding clogging and lessening aggravation!
- Skin and Hair Savior: Vitamin A and cancer prevention agents offer assistance diminish skin break out, advance solid skin, and fortify hair follicles!

Creative Ways to enjoy: Mango Franticness!

Prepared to go mango frantic? Attempt these imaginative ways to appreciate:

- Mango Salsa: Dice mango and blend with ruddy onion, jalapeño, cilantro, and lime juice for a sweet and fiery salsa!
- Mango Lassi: Mix mango, yoghourt, and drain for a velvety and reviving Indian-inspired drink!
- Mango and Avocado Serving of mixed greens: Combine diced mango, avocado, ruddy onion, and cilantro for a new and sound serving of mixed greens!

- Mango Chutney: Cook down mango with flavors and vinegar to form a sweet and tart condiment culminate for snacking or as a side dish!

There you've got it; Mango, the tropical allurement that's beyond any doubt to tempt your taste buds and feed your body! Whether you appreciate it as a nibble, include it to your top choice formulas, or utilize it as a characteristic cure, Mango is beyond any doubt to bring a burst of enhance and bliss to your life!

Orange

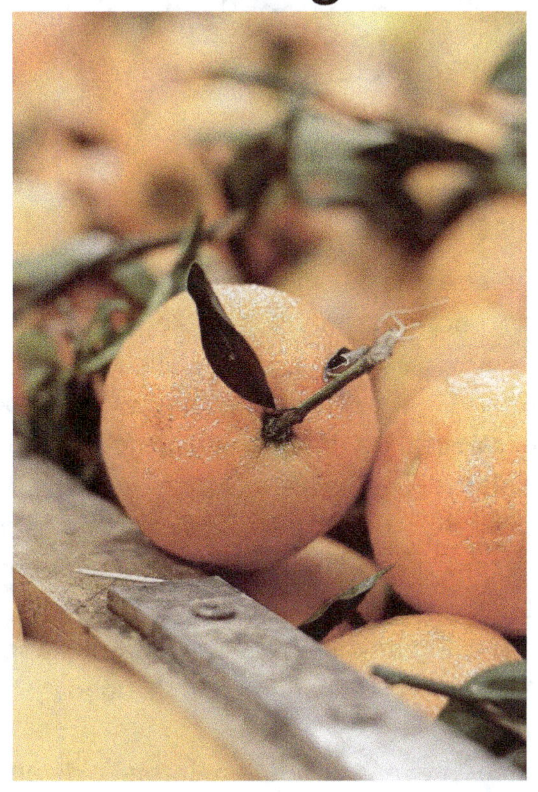

Orange: The Sunshine in Your Hands

Dietary Profile: The Juice on Orange

Meet Orange, the daylight in your hands! This dynamic, succulent charm is packed with:

- Vitamin C: 100% of your everyday needs per medium orange (that's a whopping dosage of resistance!)
- Vitamin A: 10% of your day by day needs per medium orange (supporting solid vision and resistant work)
- Fiber: 2.9 grams per medium orange (keeping your stomach related framework upbeat and sound)
- Cancer prevention agents: Carotenoids and flavonoids (battling free radicals and aggravation)

Health Benefits: The Peel-fect Bundle

So, what does this sunny genius do for you? Orange's amazing resume incorporates:

- Insusceptibility Boost: Vitamin C and cancer prevention agents offer assistance battle off contaminations and keep your resistant framework solid!
- Eye Wellbeing: Vitamin A and cancer prevention agents bolster sound vision and diminish the hazard of age-related macular degeneration! - Heart Wellbeing: Fiber, potassium, and cancer prevention agents offer assistance lower cholesterol and blood weight, keeping your heart upbeat and solid!
- Skin and Hair Savior: Vitamin C and cancer prevention agents offer assistance decrease skin break out, advance solid skin, and reinforce hair follicles!

Creative Ways to enjoy: Orange You Happy?

Prepared to urge your orange on? Attempt these inventive ways to appreciate:

- Orange and Fennel Serving of mixed greens: Combine cut oranges, fennel, and arugula for a new and solid serving of mixed greens!
- Orange and Dim Chocolate Truffles: Blend orange pizzazz and juice with dissolved dim chocolate for a debauched treat!

- Orange and Ginger Preserves: Cook down oranges with ginger and sugar for a tart and sweet spread!
- Orange and Cinnamon Water: Implant cut oranges and cinnamon sticks in water for a reviving and healthy drink!

There you have got it; Orange, the daylight in your hands that's beyond any doubt to brighten up your day! Whether you appreciate it as a nibble, include it to your favorite formulas, or utilize it as a common cure, Orange is beyond any doubt to bring a burst of flavor and delight to your life!

Watermelon

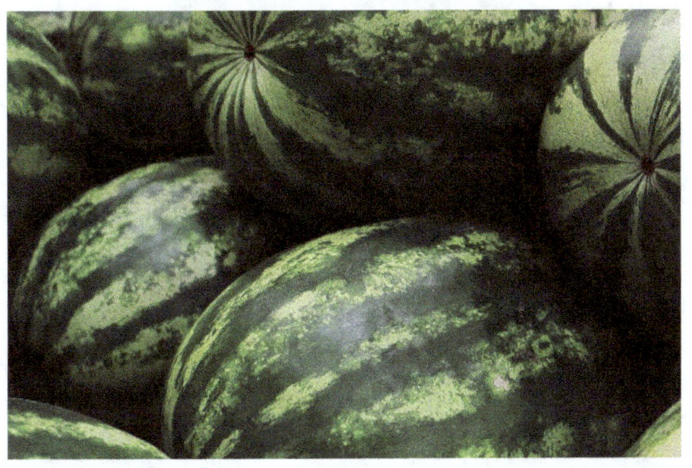

Watermelon: The Refreshing Rock star

Dietary Profile: The Juice on Watermelon

Meet Watermelon, the reviving rock star of the fruit world! This sweet, delicious charm is filled with:

- Water substance: 92% (making it one of the foremost hydrating fruits around!)
- Vitamin C: 10% of your everyday needs per container (supporting safe work and collagen generation)
- Lycopene: A effective antioxidant that battles free radicals and aggravation
- Potassium: 10% of your everyday needs per glass (making a difference direct blood weight and heart wellbeing)

Wellbeing Benefits: The Cool Stuff

So, what does this reviving rock star do for you? Watermelon's amazing resume incorporates:

- Hydration Station: Watermelon's tall water substance makes it a culminate nibble for hot summer days or post-workout refreshment!

- Antioxidant Powerhouse: Lycopene and vitamin C group up to battle free radicals and decrease irritation!
- Heart Wellbeing: Potassium and cancer prevention agents offer assistance lower blood weight and cholesterol, keeping your heart upbeat and sound!
- Skin and Hair Savior: Vitamin C and cancer prevention agents offer assistance decrease skin break out, advance solid skin, and fortify hair follicles!

Creative Ways to enjoy: Watermelon Ponder

Prepared to induce your watermelon on? Attempt these imaginative ways to appreciate:

- Watermelon and Feta Serving of mixed greens: Combine diced watermelon, feta cheese, mint, and balsamic coat for a reviving summer serving of mixed greens!
- Watermelon and Cucumber Juice: Mix watermelon, cucumber, and lime juice for a hydrating and sound drink!
- Watermelon and Berry Smoothie: Blend watermelon, solidified berries, and yoghourt for a sweet and reviving smoothie!

- Watermelon Salsa: Dice watermelon and blend
  with ruddy onion, jalapeño, cilantro, and lime
  juice for a sweet and spicy salsa!

There you've got it; Watermelon, the reviving rock
star that's beyond any doubt to extinguish your
thirst and feed your body! Whether you appreciate
it as a nibble, include it to your top pick formulas,
or utilize it as a normal cure, Watermelon is
beyond any doubt to bring a burst of enhance and
bliss to your life!

Grapes

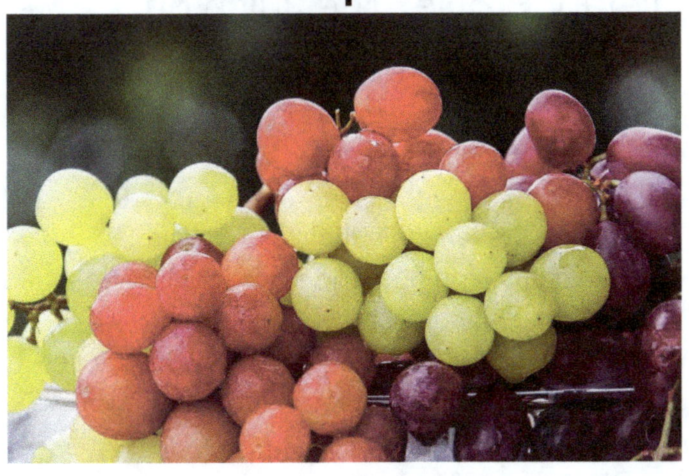

Grapes: The Tiny Titans of Taste

Dietary Profile: The Juice on Grapes

Meet Grapes, the modest titans of taste! These little, circular ponders are filled with:

- Cancer prevention agents: Resveratrol, flavonoids, and phenolic acids (battling free radicals and irritation)
- Vitamin C: 10% of your day by day needs per container (supporting resistant work and collagen generation)
- Potassium: 8% of your everyday needs per container (making a difference control blood weight and heart wellbeing)
- Fiber: 1 gram per container (supporting sound absorption and satiety)

Wellbeing Benefits: The Crush-worthy Stuff

So, what do these little titans do for you? Grapes' noteworthy resume incorporates:

- Heart Wellbeing: Cancer prevention agents and potassium offer assistance lower blood weight and cholesterol, keeping your heart cheerful and solid!
- Brain Control: Resveratrol and cancer prevention agents back cognitive work and decrease the hazard of age-related cognitive decrease!
- Anti-Inflammatory Genius: Cancer prevention agents and polyphenols decrease aggravation and battle off persistent infections!
- Skin and Hair Savior: Vitamin C and cancer prevention agents offer assistance decrease skin break out, advance solid skin, and fortify hair follicles!

Creative Ways to enjoy: Grape Desires

Prepared to urge your grape on? Attempt these inventive ways to appreciate:

- Grape and Brie Crostini: Best toasted baguette cuts with grape stick, brie cheese, and new thyme for a sweet and appetizing tidbit!
- Grape and Spinach Serving of mixed greens: Combine ruddy grapes, new spinach, disintegrated feta, and balsamic vinaigrette for a sound and reviving serving of mixed greens!

- Grape and Dim Chocolate Truffles: Blend grape juice and softened dull chocolate for a debauched and liberal treat!
- Grape and Rosemary Spritzer: Implant shimmering water with grape juice and rosemary for a reviving

Strawberry

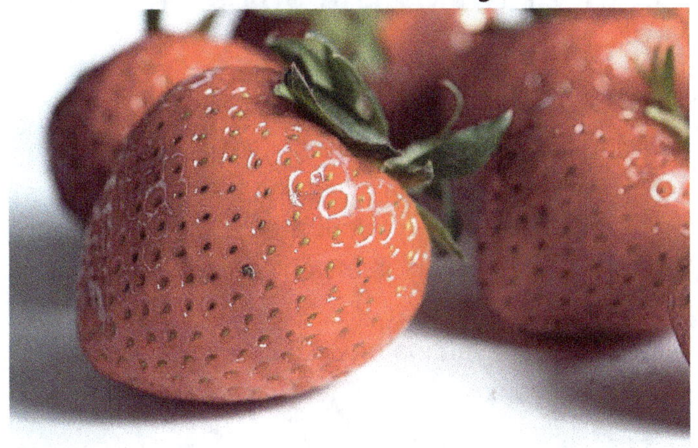

Strawberry: The Sweetheart of Fruits

Dietary Profile: The Juice on Strawberry

Meet Strawberry, the sweetheart of fruits! These delicious, ruddy delights are stuffed with:

- Vitamin C: 150% of your day by day needs per glass (supporting safe work and collagen generation)
- Cancer prevention agents: Ellagic corrosive, anthocyanin, and vitamin C (battling free radicals and aggravation)
- Fiber: 3 grams per container (supporting sound absorption and satiety)
- Potassium: 10% of your everyday needs per glass (making a difference direct blood weight and heart wellbeing)

Health Benefits: The Berry Best Stuff

So, what does this sweet whiz do for you? Strawberry's noteworthy resume incorporates:

-   Heart Wellbeing: Cancer prevention agents and potassium offer assistance lower blood weight and cholesterol, keeping your heart upbeat and sound!
-   Anti-Inflammatory Genius: Cancer prevention agents and polyphenols decrease aggravation and battle off persistent maladies!
-   Cancer Warrior: Ellagic corrosive and anthocyanin have been appeared to have anti-cancer properties!
-   Skin and Hair Savior: Vitamin C and cancer prevention agents offer assistance diminish skin break out, advance solid skin, and reinforce hair follicles!

Creative Ways to enjoy: Strawberry Splendor

Prepared to induce your strawberry on? Attempt these imaginative ways to appreciate:

-   Strawberry and Spinach Serving of mixed greens: Combine fresh strawberries, infant spinach, feta cheese, and balsamic vinaigrette for a sound and reviving serving of mixed greens!
-   Strawberry and Dim Chocolate Fondue: Plunge new strawberries, bananas, and pineapple cuts

in softened dim chocolate for a debauched treat!
- Strawberry and Mint Smoothie: Mix fresh strawberries, mint clears out, yoghourt, and nectar for a sweet and reviving smoothie!
- Strawberry and Balsamic Coat: Sprinkle balsamic coat over fresh strawberries and whipped cream for a sweet and tangy dessert!

There you have got it; Strawberry, the sweetheart of fruits that's beyond any doubt to capture your heart with its sweet enhance and noteworthy nourishment! Whether you appreciate them as a nibble, include them to your top choice formulas, or utilize them as a common cure, Strawberries are beyond any doubt to bring a burst of enhance and delight to your life!

Pineapple

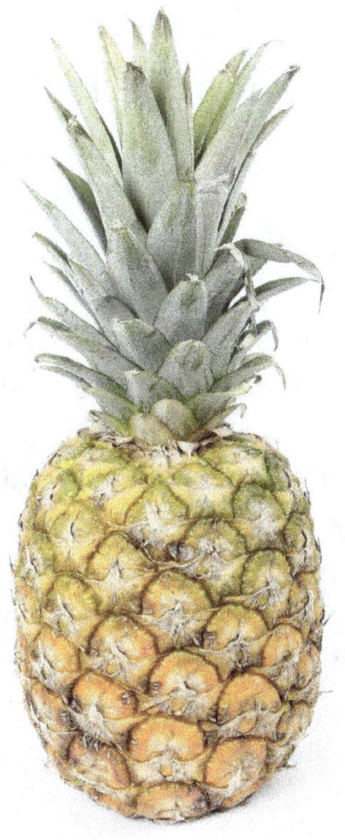

Pineapple: The Tropical Temptress

Wholesome Profile: The Juice on Pineapple

Meet Pineapple, the tropical flirt! This sweet, tart, and delicious charm is stuffed with:

- Vitamin C: 131% of your everyday needs per container (supporting safe work and collagen generation)
- Manganese: 76% of your everyday needs per container (supporting bone wellbeing and digestion system)
- Cancer prevention agents: Different polyphenols and flavonoids (battling free radicals and irritation)
- Fiber: 2.3 grams per container (supporting sound assimilation and satiety)

Health Benefits: The Island of Wellness

So, what does this tropical flirt do for you? Pineapple's amazing resume incorporates:

- Insusceptibility Boost: Vitamin C and cancer prevention agents offer assistance battle off diseases and keep your resistant framework solid!
- Anti-Inflammatory Genius: Cancer prevention agents and polyphenols diminish aggravation and battle off persistent illnesses!
- Stomach related Enchant: Fiber and cancer prevention agents bolster sound absorption and decrease indications of IBS!
- Cancer Warrior: Different cancer prevention agents and polyphenols have been appeared to have anti-cancer properties!

Creative Ways to enjoy: Pineapple Rise

Prepared to urge your pineapple on? Attempt these imaginative ways to appreciate:

- Pineapple and Coconut Smoothie: Mix new pineapple, coconut drain, and a imply of lime for a tropical treat!
- Pineapple and Ham Pizza: Beat a hand crafted pizza outside with pineapple rings, ham cuts, and mozzarella cheese for a sweet and exquisite charm!
- Pineapple and Mango Salsa: Combine diced pineapple, mango, ruddy onion, jalapeño,

cilantro, and lime juice for a sweet and hot salsa!
- Pineapple and Ginger Jelly: Cook down new pineapple and ginger for a tart and sweet spread culminate for toast or yoghourt!

There you've got it; Pineapple, the tropical seductress that's beyond any doubt to transport you to an island of wellness and enhance! Whether you appreciate it as a nibble, include it to your top pick formulas, or utilize it as a normal cure, Pineapple is beyond any doubt to bring a burst of enhance and bliss to your life!

Peach

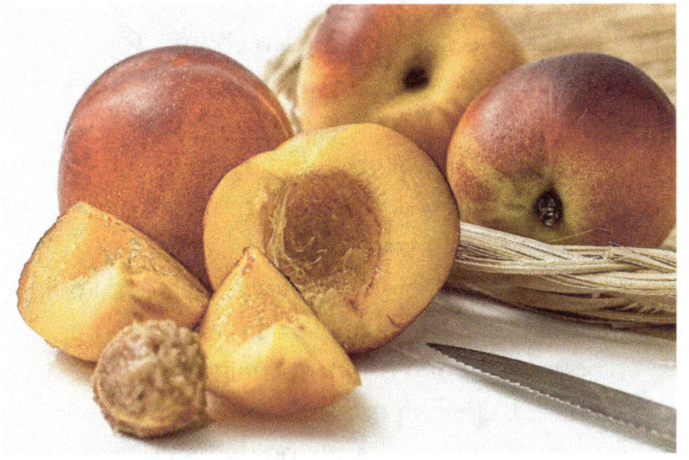

Peach: The Sweet Southern Charm

Dietary Profile: The Juice on Peach

Meet Peach, the sweet southern charm! This succulent, sweet, and juicy charm is stuffed with:

- Vitamin C: 10% of your day by day needs per medium peach (supporting safe work and collagen generation)
- Potassium: 8% of your day by day needs per medium peach (making a difference control blood weight and heart wellbeing)
- Fiber: 2.5 grams per medium peach (supporting solid absorption and satiety)
- Cancer prevention agents: Different polyphenols and flavonoids (battling free radicals and aggravation)

Wellbeing Benefits: The Peachy Sharp Stuff

So, what does this sweet southern charm do for you? Peach's amazing resume incorporates:

- Heart Wellbeing: Potassium and cancer prevention agents offer assistance lower blood

weight and cholesterol, keeping your heart
upbeat and sound!
- Anti-Inflammatory Whiz: Cancer prevention
agents and polyphenols diminish aggravation
and battle off unremitting maladies!
- Stomach related Charm: Fiber and cancer
prevention agents bolster solid absorption and
decrease indications of IBS!
- Skin and Hair Savior: Vitamin C and cancer
prevention agents offer assistance diminish
skin break out, advance sound skin, and fortify
hair follicles!

Creative Ways to enjoy: Peachy Sharp Thoughts

Prepared to urge your peach on? Attempt these
imaginative ways to appreciate:

- Peach and Brie Serving of mixed greens:
Combine cut peaches, brie cheese, blended
greens, and balsamic vinaigrette for a sweet
and savory serving of mixed greens!
- Peach and Ginger Smoothie: Mix new
peaches, ginger, yogurt, and nectar for a sweet
and reviving smoothie!
- Peach and Prosciutto Pizza: Beat a hand
crafted pizza outside with peach cuts,

prosciutto, and mozzarella cheese for a sweet and salty charm!

- Peach and Cinnamon Cereal: Include cut peaches and cinnamon to your oats for a warm and comforting breakfast!

There you have got it; Peach, the sweet southern charm that's beyond any doubt to capture your heart with its sweet flavor and amazing nourishment! Whether you appreciate it as a nibble, include it to your favorite formulas, or utilize it as a common cure, Peach is beyond any doubt to bring a burst of flavor and bliss to your life!

Cherry

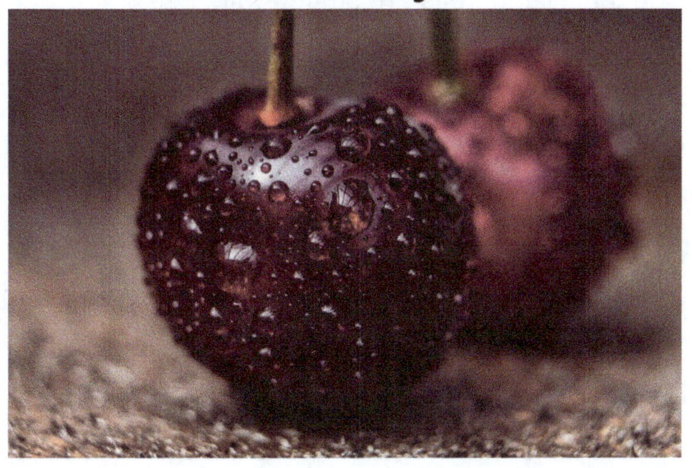

Cherry: The Juicy Jewel

Dietary Profile: The Juice on Cherry

Meet Cherry, the delicious gem! These stout, tart, and tantalizing fruits are stuffed with:

- Cancer prevention agents: Quercetin, anthocyanin, and vitamin C (battling free radicals and aggravation)
- Fiber: 3 grams per glass (supporting sound absorption and satiety)
- Vitamin C: 10% of your everyday needs per container (supporting resistant work and collagen generation)
- Potassium: 10% of your everyday needs per container (making a difference direct blood weight and heart wellbeing)

Wellbeing Benefits: The Cherry on Beat

So, what does this delicious gem do for you? Cherry's amazing resume incorporates:

- Heart Wellbeing: Cancer prevention agents and potassium offer assistance to lower blood

weight and cholesterol, keeping your heart cheerful and solid!
- Anti-Inflammatory Whiz: Cancer prevention agents and polyphenols decrease aggravation and battle off inveterate maladies!
- Rest Savior: Cherry juice has appeared to progress to rest quality and term!
- Torment Alleviation: Cherry juice has anti-inflammatory properties that will offer assistance to diminish muscle and joint torment!

Creative Ways to enjoy: Cherry-O Thoughts

Prepared to urge your cherry on? Attempt these imaginative ways to appreciate:

- Cherry and Chocolate Fondue: Plunge new cherries, strawberries, and pineapple cuts in liquefied dull chocolate for a debauched treat!
- Cherry and Almond Smoothie: Mix new cherries, almond drain, and a dash of vanilla for a sweet and reviving smoothie!
- Cherry and Brie Barbecued Cheese: Beat a barbecued cheese sandwich with cherry stick and brie cheese for a sweet and savory enchant!

- Cherry and Coconut Cereal: Include dried cherries and destroyed coconut to your cereal for a warm and comforting breakfast!

There you have got it; Cherry, the succulent gem that's beyond any doubt to include a burst of flavor and nourishment to your life! Whether you appreciate it as a nibble, include it in your favorite formulas, or utilize it as a natural remedy, Cherry is sure to bring a grin to your confrontation!

Pomegranate

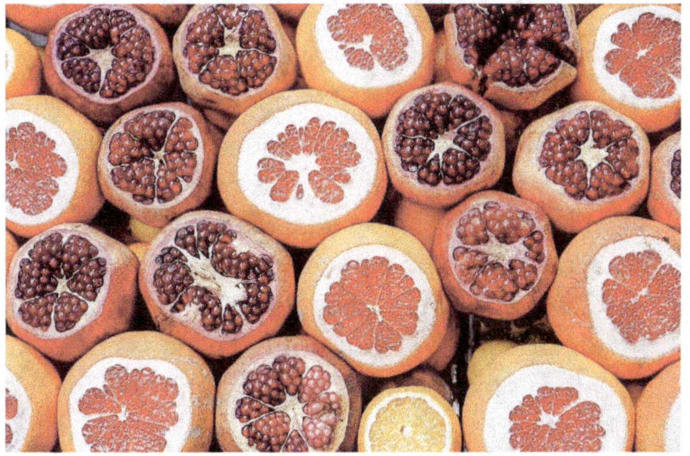

Pomegranate: The Ruby Red Rock star

Dietary Profile: The Juice on Pomegranate

Meet Pomegranate, the ruby ruddy rock star! This succulent, tart, and tempting fruit is filled with:

- Cancer prevention agents: Ellagic corrosive, punicalagins, and anthocyanin (battling free radicals and aggravation)
- Vitamin C: 16% of your everyday needs per container (supporting safe work and collagen generation)
- Potassium: 12% of your everyday needs per container (making a difference control blood weight and heart wellbeing)
- Fiber: 4 grams per glass (supporting sound absorption and satiety)

Health Benefits: The Pomegranate Powerhouse

So, what does this ruby ruddy rock star do for you? Pomegranate's amazing resume incorporates:

- Heart Wellbeing: Cancer prevention agents and potassium offer assistance to lower blood weight and cholesterol, keeping your heart cheerful and sound!
- Anti-Inflammatory Whiz: Cancer prevention agents and polyphenols decrease aggravation and battle off persistent illnesses!
- Anti-Cancer Properties: Ellagic corrosive and punicalagins have been shown to have anti-cancer properties!
- Brain Control: Pomegranate juice has appeared to make strides in memory and cognitive work!

Creative Ways to enjoy: Pomegranate Palooza

Prepared to urge your pomegranate on? Attempt these imaginative ways to appreciate:

- Pomegranate and Avocado Serving of mixed greens: Combine blended greens, diced pomegranate, avocado, and a citrus vinaigrette for a solid and reviving serving of mixed greens!
- Pomegranate and Dull Chocolate Truffles: Blend pomegranate juice and dissolved dull chocolate for a debauched and liberal treat!

- Pomegranate and Quinoa Bowl: Beat cooked quinoa with diced pomegranate, broiled vegetables, and a dab of yoghurt for a nutritious and filling bowl!
- Pomegranate and Ginger Jelly: Cook down pomegranate juice and ginger for a tart and sweet spread culminates for toast or yoghurt!

There you have it; Pomegranate, the ruby ruddy rock star that's beyond any doubt to include a burst of enhancement and sustenance to your life! Whether you appreciate it as a nibble, include it to your top choice formulas, or utilize it as a natural remedy, Pomegranate is beyond any doubt to bring a grin to your confrontation!

Acai berry

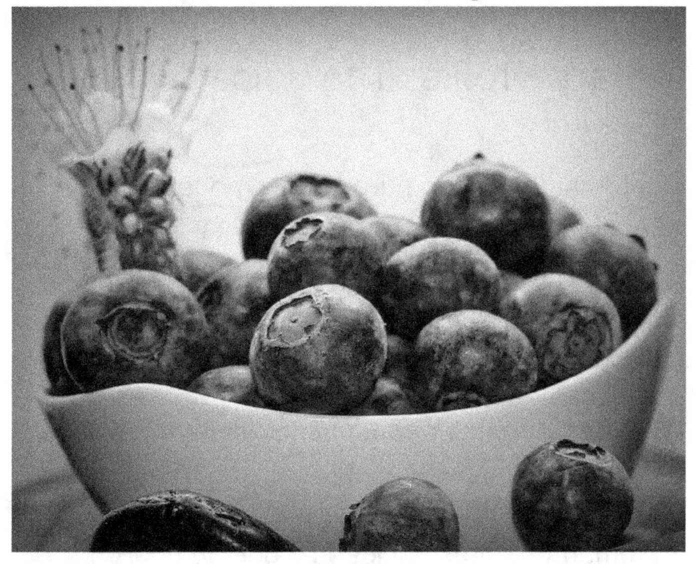

Acai Berry: The Purple Powerhouse

Dietary Profile: The Juice on Acai Berry

Meet Acai Berry, the purple powerhouse! These little, dull purple fruits are stuffed with:

- Cancer prevention agents: Anthocyanin, polyphenols, and vitamin C (battling free radicals and irritation)
- Fiber: 4 grams per container (supporting sound assimilation and satiety)
- Heart-healthy fats: Omega-3, omega-6, and omega-9 greasy acids (supporting heart wellbeing and brain work)
- Vitamins and minerals: Vitamin A, vitamin C, potassium, and magnesium (supporting resistant work, eye wellbeing, and vitality generation)

Health Benefits: The Acai Advantage

So, what does this purple powerhouse do for you? Acai Berry noteworthy resume incorporates:

- Heart Wellbeing: Cancer prevention agents, fiber, and heart-healthy fats offer assistance to lower cholesterol and blood weight, keeping your heart cheerful and solid!
- Anti-Inflammatory Whiz: Cancer prevention agents and polyphenols diminish aggravation and battle off inveterate maladies!
- Brain Control: Omega-3 greasy acids and cancer prevention agents back brain work, memory, and cognitive wellbeing!
- Insusceptibility Boost: Vitamin C, vitamin A, and cancer prevention agents back safe work and diminish the hazard of ailments!

Creative Ways to enjoy: Acai Berry Euphoria

Prepared to urge your acai on? Attempt these inventive ways to appreciate:

- Acai and Banana Smoothie: Mix solidified acai berries, banana, almond drain, and nectar for a sweet and reviving smoothie!
- Acai and Granola Bowl: Beat cooked oats or quinoa with acai berries, granola, and fresh fruits for a nutritious and filling breakfast!
- Acai and Dim Chocolate Truffles: Blend acai berry powder and liquefied dull chocolate for a debauched and liberal treat!

- Acai and Coconut Water Refresher: Imbue coconut water with acai berry powder and a crush of lime for a reviving and healthy drink!

There you have got it; Acai Berry, the purple powerhouse that's beyond any doubt to include a burst of flavor and nourishment to your life! Whether you appreciate it as a nibble, include it in your favorite formulas, or utilize it as a characteristic cure, Acai Berry is beyond any doubt to bring a grin to your confrontation!

Blueberries

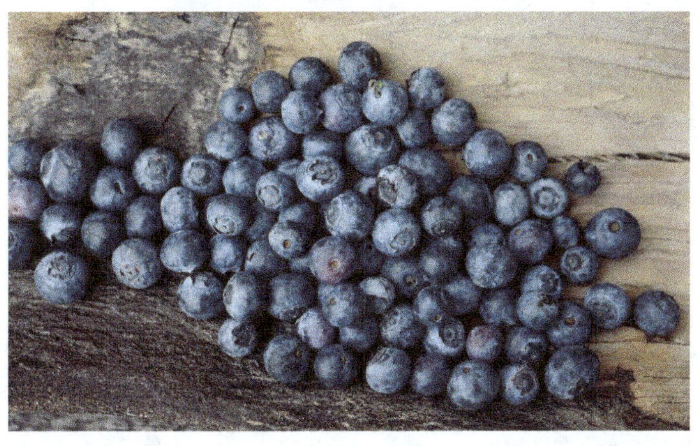

Blueberries: The Tiny Titans of Taste

Dietary Profile: The Juice on Blueberries

Meet Blueberries, the little titans of taste! These little, circular ponders are packed with:

- Cancer prevention agents: Anthocyanin, polyphenols, and vitamin C (battling free radicals and aggravation)
- Fiber: 4 grams per container (supporting solid absorption and satiety)
- Brain-healthy compounds: Flavonoids and phenolic acids (supporting cognitive work and memory)
- Vitamins and minerals: Vitamin C, vitamin K, potassium, and manganese (supporting resistant work, bone wellbeing, and vitality generation)

Health Benefits: The Blueberry Boost

So, what do these modest titans do for you?

Blueberries' noteworthy resume incorporates:

- Brain Control: Flavonoids and phenolic acids bolster cognitive work, memory, and center!
- Heart Wellbeing: Cancer prevention agents, fiber, and potassium offer assistance lower cholesterol and blood weight, keeping your heart upbeat and solid!
- Anti-Inflammatory Whiz: Cancer prevention agents and polyphenols diminish aggravation and battle off constant maladies!
- Resistance Boost: Vitamin C, vitamin K, and cancer prevention agents back safe work and decrease the hazard of sicknesses!

Creative Ways to enjoy: Blueberry Rapture

Prepared to urge your blueberry on? Attempt these inventive ways to appreciate:

- Blueberry and Greek Yoghourts Parfait: Layer Greek yoghurt, fresh blueberries, and granola for a protein.

Raspberry

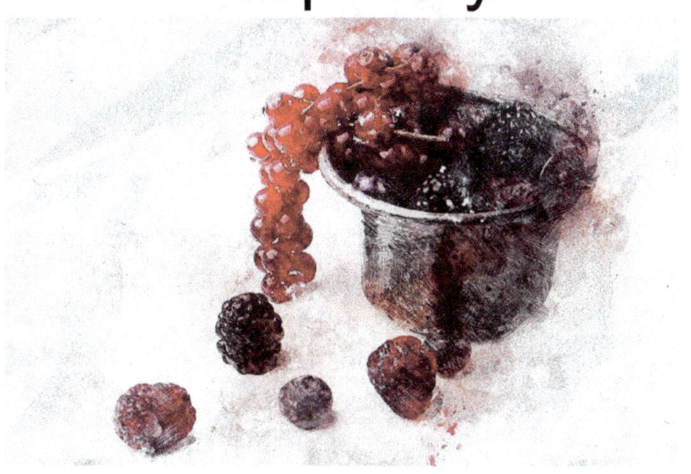

Raspberry: The Ruby Red Rock star

Dietary Profile: The Juice on Raspberry

Meet Raspberry, the ruby ruddy rockstar! These sweet-tart ponders are filled with:

- Cancer prevention agents: Ellagic corrosive, anthocyanin, and vitamin C (battling free radicals and irritation)
- Fiber: 4 grams per glass (supporting solid assimilation and satiety)
- Vitamins and minerals: Vitamin C, vitamin K, potassium, and manganese (supporting safe work, bone wellbeing, and vitality generation) - Heart-healthy compounds: Flavonoids and phenolic acids (supporting cardiovascular wellbeing)

Health Benefits: The Raspberry Rave

So, what does this ruby ruddy rockstar do for you? Raspberry's noteworthy resume incorporates:

- Heart Wellbeing: Cancer prevention agents, fiber, and heart-healthy compounds offer

assistance to lower cholesterol and blood weight, keeping your heart upbeat and solid!
- Anti-Inflammatory Genius: Cancer prevention agents and polyphenols diminish irritation and battle off constant illnesses!
- Resistance Boost: Vitamin C, vitamin K, and cancer prevention agents back safe work and decrease the chance of ailments!
- Cancer Warrior: Ellagic corrosive and anthocyanin have been shown to have anti-cancer properties!

Creative Ways to enjoy: Raspberry Composition

Prepared to urge your raspberry on? Attempt these inventive ways to appreciate:

- Raspberry and Chocolate Chip Cereal: Include new raspberries and dim chocolate chips to your oats for a sweet and fulfilling breakfast!
- Raspberry and Brie Flame broiled Cheese: Best a flame broiled cheese sandwich with raspberry stick and brie cheese for a sweet and appetizing enchant!
- Raspberry and Lemonade Refresher: Implant lemonade with new raspberries and a sprig of mint for a reviving summer drink!
- Raspberry and Dull Chocolate Truffles: Blend raspberry stick and dissolved dim chocolate for a wanton and indulgent treat!

There you have it; Raspberry, the ruby ruddy rock star that's beyond any doubt to include a burst of enhancement and sustenance to your life! Whether you appreciate them as a nibble, include them to your top pick formulas, or utilize them as a common cure, Raspberries are beyond any doubt to bring a grin to your confrontation!

Lemon

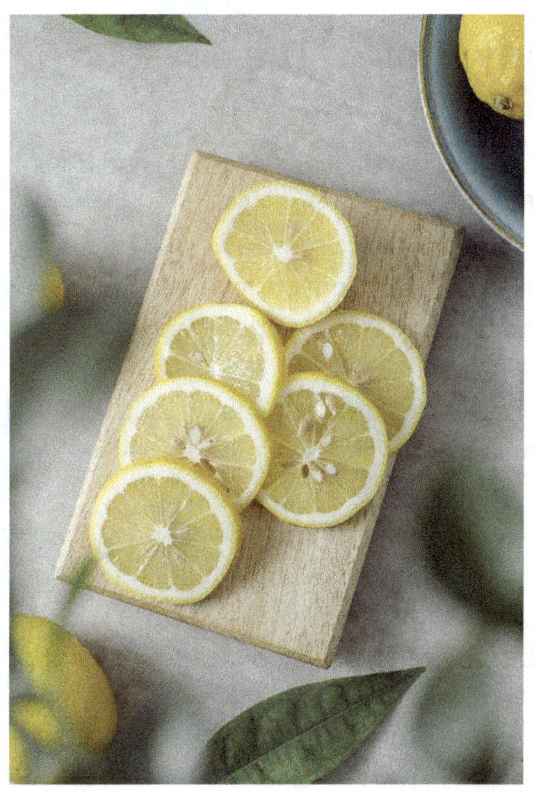

Lemon: The Sunshine Superstar

Dietary Profile: The Juice on Lemon

Meet Lemon, the daylight whiz! This shining and cheerful citrus fruit is stuffed with:

- Vitamin C: 53% of your everyday needs per medium lemon (supporting resistant work and collagen generation)
- Cancer prevention agents: Flavonoids and limuloids (battling free radicals and aggravation)
- Potassium: 8% of your day by day needs per medium lemon (making a difference control blood weight and heart wellbeing)
- Fiber: 2 grams per medium lemon (supporting solid assimilation and satiety)

Health Benefits: The Lemon Adore

So, what does this daylight whiz do for you? Lemon's noteworthy resume incorporates:

- Resistance Boost: Vitamin C and cancer prevention agents bolster resistant work and decrease the chance of ailments!

- Heart Wellbeing: Potassium and cancer prevention agents offer assistance to lower blood weight and cholesterol, keeping your heart upbeat and solid!
- Anti-Inflammatory Genius: Cancer prevention agents and flavonoids decrease irritation and battle off persistent illnesses!
- Stomach related Charm: Fiber and cancer prevention agents back solid assimilation and decrease side effects of IBS!

Creative Ways to enjoy: Lemon Adore Issue

Prepared to induce your lemon on? Attempt these imaginative ways to appreciate:

- Lemon and Ginger Zinger: Implant water with new lemon and ginger for a reviving and solid drink!
- Lemon and Herb Simmered Chicken: Marinate chicken with lemon juice, olive oil, and herbs for a flavorful and sodden dish!
- Lemon and Berry Serving of mixed greens: Combine blended greens, new berries, and a crush of lemon for a light and reviving serving of mixed greens!
- Lemon and Dull Chocolate Truffles: Blend lemon pizazz and liquefied dull chocolate for a tart and indulgent treat!

There you have got it; Lemon, the daylight whiz that's beyond any doubt to include a burst of enhancement and nourishment to your life! Whether you appreciate it as a nibble, include it to your top pick formulas, or utilize it as a normal cure, Lemon is beyond any doubt to bring a grin to your confrontation!

Kiwi

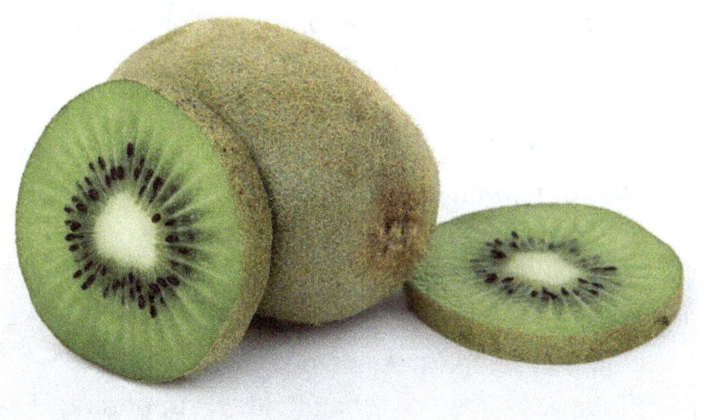

Kiwi: The Tiny Titan of Taste

Dietary Profile: The Juice on Kiwi

Meet Kiwi, the modest titan of taste! This little, textured natural product is stuffed with:

- Vitamin C: 70% of your everyday needs per medium kiwi (supporting safe work and collagen generation)
- Potassium: 10% of your everyday needs per medium kiwi (making a difference direct blood weight and heart wellbeing)
- Fiber: 2 grams per medium kiwi (supporting sound assimilation and satiety)
- Cancer prevention agents: Polyphenols and carotenoids (battling free radicals and aggravation)

Health Benefits: The Kiwi Kick

So, what does this minor titan do for you? Kiwi's amazing resume incorporates:

- Insusceptibility Boost: Vitamin C and cancer prevention agents back safe work and diminish the chance of sicknesses!

- Heart Wellbeing: Potassium and cancer prevention agents offer assistance to lower blood weight and cholesterol, keeping your heart upbeat and sound!
- Anti-Inflammatory Genius: Cancer prevention agents and polyphenols diminish irritation and battle off inveterate infections!
- Stomach related Charm: Fiber and cancer prevention agents bolster solid absorption and decrease indications of IBS!

Creative Ways to enjoy: Kiwi Fever

Prepared to induce your kiwi on? Attempt these inventive ways to appreciate:

- Kiwi and Strawberry Smoothie: Mix kiwi, strawberry, and yoghurt for a sweet and reviving smoothie!
- Kiwi and Avocado Salsa: Combine diced kiwi, avocado, ruddy onion, and jalapeño for a new and zesty salsa!
- Kiwi and Flame broiled Chicken Serving of mixed greens: Best blended greens with flame broiled chicken, cut kiwi, and a citrus vinaigrette for a sound and flavorful serving of mixed greens!
- Kiwi and Coconut Cream Pie: Blend kiwi puree with coconut cream and lime juice for a velvety and indulgent dessert!

There you have got it; Kiwi, the modest titan of taste that's beyond any doubt to include a burst of enhancement and sustenance to your life! Whether you appreciate it as a nibble, include it to your top pick formulas, or utilize it as a characteristic cure, Kiwi is beyond any doubt to bring a grin to your confrontation!

Papaya

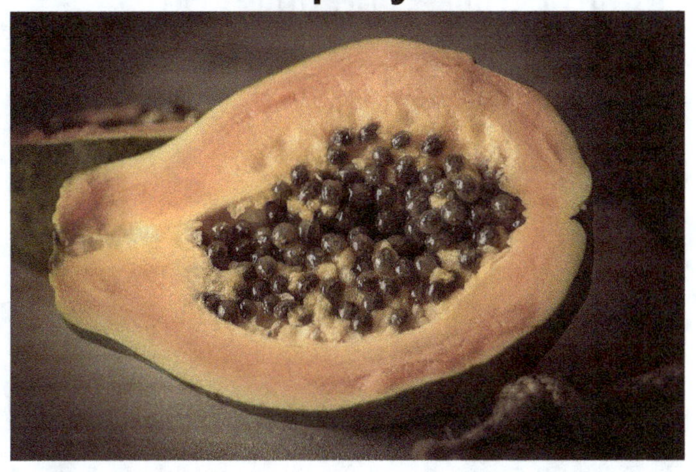

Papaya: The Tropical Temptress

Health Profile: The Juice on Papaya

Meet Papaya, the tropical flirt! This delicious, orange-pink fruit is packed with:

- Vitamin C: 100% of your day by day needs per medium papaya (supporting resistant work and collagen generation)
- Potassium: 11% of your day by day needs per medium papaya (making a difference control blood weight and heart wellbeing)
- Fiber: 2.5 grams per medium papaya (supporting sound assimilation and satiety)
- Cancer prevention agents: Lycopene and polyphenols (battling free radicals and irritation)

Health Benefits: The Papaya Heaven

So, what does this tropical flirt do for you? Papaya's amazing continue incorporates:

- Insusceptibility Boost: Vitamin C and cancer prevention agents bolster safe work and diminish the hazard of ailments!

- Heart Wellbeing: Potassium and cancer prevention agents offer assistance to lower blood weight and cholesterol, keeping your heart upbeat and solid!
- Anti-Inflammatory Whiz: Cancer prevention agents and lycopene decrease irritation and battle off incessant infections!
- Stomach related Enchant: Fiber and cancer prevention agents back solid absorption and decrease indications of IBS!

Creative Ways to enjoy: Papaya Energy

Prepared to urge your papaya on? Attempt these imaginative ways to appreciate:

- Papaya and Mango Salsa: Combine diced papaya, mango, ruddy onion, and jalapeño for a new and hot salsa!
- Papaya and Coconut Smoothie: Mix papaya, coconut drain, and an indication of lime for a velvety and reviving smoothie!
- Papaya and Flame broiled Chicken Serving of mixed greens: Best blended greens with flame broiled chicken, cut papaya, and a citrus vinaigrette for a solid and flavorful serving of mixed greens!
- Papaya and Pineapple Upside-Down Cake: Blend papaya puree with pineapple rings and

an impl of cinnamon for a sweet and indulgent dessert!

There you've got it; Papaya, the tropical seductress that's beyond any doubt to include a burst of enhancement and sustenance to your life! Whether you appreciate it as a nibble, include it to your top choice formulas, or utilize it as a common cure, Papaya is beyond any doubt to bring a grin to your confrontation!

Guava

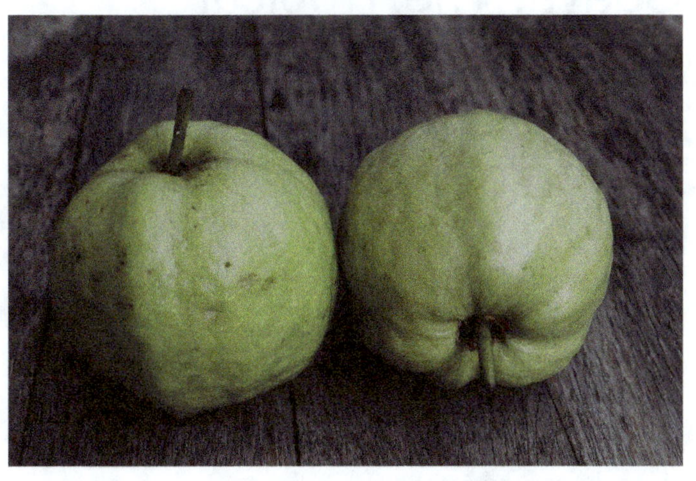

Guava: The Tropical Sweetheart

Dietary Profile: The Juice on Guava

Meet Guava, the tropical sweetheart! This dynamic, pink or yellow fruit is packed with:

- Vitamin C: 250% of your day by day needs per medium guava (supporting safe work and collagen generation)
- Cancer prevention agents: Lycopene, flavonoids, and polyphenols (battling free radicals and irritation)
- Fiber: 5 grams per medium guava (supporting sound absorption and satiety)
- Potassium: 10% of your day by day needs per medium guava (making a difference control blood weight and heart wellbeing)

Health Benefits: The Guava Gleam

So, what does this tropical sweetheart do for you? Guava's amazing continue incorporates:

- Resistance Boost: Vitamin C and cancer prevention agents back safe work and diminish the hazard of ailments!

- Anti-Inflammatory Genius: Cancer prevention agents and lycopene diminish aggravation and battle off incessant infections!
- Heart Wellbeing: Potassium and cancer prevention agents offer assistance to lower blood weight and cholesterol, keeping your heart upbeat and solid!
- Stomach related Charm: Fiber and cancer prevention agents back sound absorption and diminish indications of IBS!

Creative Ways to enjoy: Guava Free for all

Prepared to urge your guava on? Attempt these inventive ways to appreciate:

- Guava and Coconut Water Refresher: Imbue coconut water with guava puree and a crush of lime for a reviving and sound drink!
- Guava and Avocado Salsa: Combine diced guava, avocado, ruddy onion, and jalapeño for a new and hot salsa!
- Guava and Flame broiled Chicken Serving of mixed greens: Best blended greens with barbecued chicken, cut guava, and a citrus vinaigrette for a solid and flavorful serving of mixed greens!
- Guava and Cream Cheese Empanadas: Blend guava puree with cream cheese and wrap in a

firm empanada outside for a sweet and indulgent dessert!

There you've got it; Guava, the tropical sweetheart that's beyond any doubt to include a burst of enhancement and sustenance to your life! Whether you appreciate it as a nibble, include it to your top pick formulas, or utilize it as a common cure, Guava is beyond any doubt to bring a grin to your confrontation!

Mangosteen

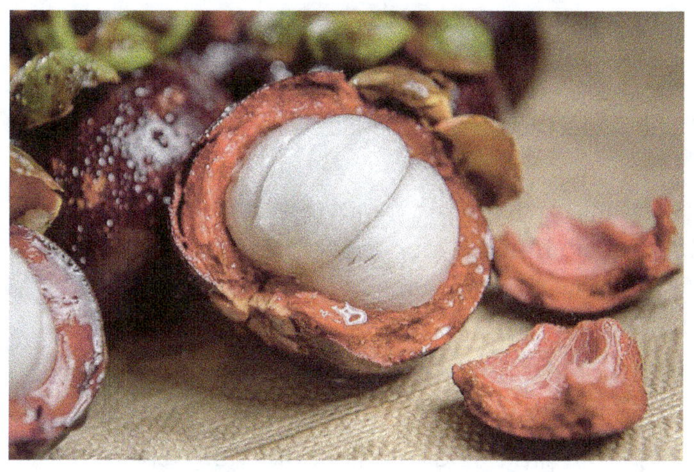

Mangosteen: The Purple Princess

Health Profile: The Juice on Mangosteen

Meet Mangosteen, the purple princess! This outlandish, purple fruit is filled with:

- Vitamin C: 45% of your everyday needs per medium mangosteen (supporting resistant work and collagen generation)
- Cancer prevention agents: Xanthones, flavonoids, and polyphenols (battling free radicals and irritation)
- Fiber: 2 grams per medium mangosteen (supporting solid assimilation and satiety)
- Potassium: 8% of your everyday needs per medium mangosteen (making a difference control blood weight and heart wellbeing)

Health Benefits: The Mangosteen Enchantment

So, what does this purple princess do for you? Mangosteen's noteworthy resume incorporates:

- Resistance Boost: Vitamin C and cancer prevention agents bolster safe work and decrease the hazard of ailments!
- Anti-Inflammatory Genius: Cancer prevention agents and xanthones diminish aggravation and battle off persistent maladies!
- Heart Wellbeing: Potassium and cancer prevention agents offer assistance to lower blood weight and cholesterol, keeping your heart upbeat and sound!
- Stomach related Enchant: Fiber and cancer prevention agents back solid assimilation and decrease side effects of IBS!

Creative Ways to enjoy: Mangosteen Lunacy

Prepared to urge your mangosteen on? Attempt these inventive ways to appreciate:

- Mangosteen and Coconut Water Refresher: Implant coconut water with mangosteen puree and a press of lime for a reviving and solid drink!
- Mangosteen and Pineapple Salsa: Combine diced mangosteen, pineapple, ruddy onion, and jalapeño for a sweet and fiery salsa!
- Mangosteen and Flame broiled Chicken Serving of mixed greens: Beat blended greens with barbecued chicken, cut mangosteen, and a

citrus vinaigrette for a solid and flavorful serving of mixed greens!

-        Mangosteen and Dull Chocolate Truffles: Blend mangosteen puree with dissolved dull chocolate and an impiety of coconut for a wanton and indulgent treat!

There you've got it; Mangosteen, the purple princess that's beyond any doubt to include a burst of flavor and sustenance to your life! Whether you appreciate it as a nibble, include it in your favorite formulas, or utilize it as a natural remedy, Mangosteen is beyond any doubt to bring a grin to your confrontation!

Dragon fruit

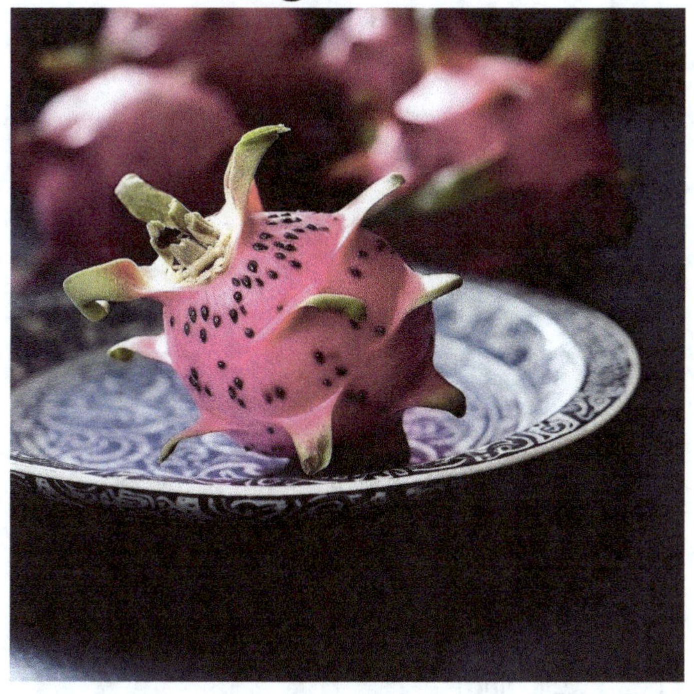

Dragon Fruit: The Vibrant Vixen

Health Profile: The Juice on Mythical Serpent Natural product

Meet Mythical beast fruit, the dynamic lady! This staggering, pink or yellow fruit is filled with:

- Vitamin C: 34% of your everyday needs per medium mythical serpent natural product (supporting safe work and collagen generation)
- Cancer prevention agents: Betalains, flavonoids, and polyphenols (battling free radicals and irritation)
- Fiber: 2.5 grams per medium mythical serpent natural product (supporting sound absorption and satiety)
- Potassium: 10% of your day by day needs per medium mythical beast natural product (making a difference direct blood weight and heart wellbeing)

Health Benefits: The Mythical Beast Natural Product Enchant

So, what does this dynamic lady do for you? Mythical beast Fruit's amazing resume incorporates:

-       Insusceptibility Boost: Vitamin C and cancer prevention agents bolster safe work and diminish the chance of ailments!

-       Anti-Inflammatory Genius: Cancer prevention agents and betalains decrease irritation and battle off constant infections!

-       Heart Wellbeing: Potassium and cancer prevention agents offer assistance to lower blood weight and cholesterol, keeping your heart cheerful and solid!

-       Stomach related Enchant: Fiber and cancer prevention agents bolster solid assimilation and diminish side effects of IBS!

Creative Ways to enjoy: Winged serpent fruit Free for all

Prepared to urge your mythical serpent fruit on? Attempt these inventive ways to enjoy:

-       Mythical serpent fruit and Coconut Water Refresher: Imbue coconut water with mythical beast fruit puree and a press of lime for a reviving and solid drink!

-       Mythical beast Natural product and Mango Salsa: Combine diced mythical serpent natural product, mango, ruddy onion, and jalapeño for a sweet and fiery salsa!

-       Winged serpent fruit and Barbecued Chicken Serving of mixed greens: Best blended greens with barbecued chicken, cut winged serpent fruit, and a citrus vinaigrette for a solid and flavorful serving of mixed greens!

-       Winged serpent fruit and Dull Chocolate Truffles: Blend mythical serpent fruit puree with liquefied dull chocolate and an imply of coconut

Incorporating Fruits into Your Daily Diet: A Delicious Path to Wellness!

Hey there, fellow enthusiast! Are you seeking ways to add more color, flavor, and nutrition to your daily diet? You're definitely in the right place! Incorporating fruits into your daily diet can have a significant impact on your general health and wellbeing. And the best part is that it's easier than you think!

Tips for Adding More Fruits to Your Daily Diet:

- Start little by little: Begin with one or two servings a day and gradually increase your intake as you improve.
- Mix and compare: Experiment with different combinations of fruit to arrive at your favorites.
- Make it convenient: Keep a bowl of different fruits on your counter or dining, and U can also pre-wash and chop the fruits for easy snacking.
- Sneak it in: include fruits to your favorite smoothies, salads, and desserts.

Fruit Portion Sizes and Serving Suggestions:

- Aim for 2-3 servings a day which is about 1-2 cups.
- It can be Fresh, frozen, or dried; all count towards your daily goal!
- Attempt these serving ideas:
- Fresh berries with oatmeal or yoghourt
- Sliced apples with almond butter
- Banana "ice cream" (freeze and blend for a creamy treat!)

Creative Ways to Enjoy Fruit:

- **Smoothies**: Blend your favourite fruits with yoghourt, milk, or ice cream for a quick and refreshing drink.
- **Salads**: Mix sliced fruits with greens, nuts, and cheese for a sweet and savory mix.
- **Desserts**: Use fruits to sweeten your treats, like baked apples or fruit-topped yoghourt parfaits!

More Ideas to Get You Started:

- Add sliced citrus to your water for a refreshing twist.
- Make a fruit and cheese platter for a healthy and refreshing snack.

- Use fruits as toppings for oatmeal, yoghurt, or even savory dishes like grilled meats or salads! Including fruits into your daily diet is an easy and delicious way to boost your health and satisfaction. So ensure to go ahead, get creative, and enjoy the fruit-filled journey!

Delicious Fruit Mixtures for Smoothies and Drinks: A Taste of Paradise!

Hello there, fellow fruit enthusiast! Are you tired of the same ancient smoothie schedule? Do you need to level up your hydration and fulfil your sweet tooth? You're within the right put! Get ready to enjoy the most delicious fruit blends that will make your taste buds move with delight!

10 Reviving Natural Product Smoothie Formulas:

1. Tropical Euphoria:
Pineapple, mango, coconut drain, and an impl of lime.
2. Berry Boost:
Blueberries, strawberries, bananas, and almonds drain.
3. Peachy Sharp:
Peaches, pineapple, orange juice, and a sprinkle of cinnamon.
4. Green Goddess:
Avocado, spinach, banana, and lemon juice.
5. Mango Franticness:
Mango, pineapple, coconut water, and a sprinkle of lime.
6. Citrus Dawn:

Orange, grapefruit, pineapple, and an indication of nectar.

7.   Antioxidant Impact:

Blueberries, raspberries, blackberries, and almond drain.

8. Pina Colada:

Pineapple, coconut drain, and a sprinkle of cinnamon.

9. Strawberry Banana Charm:

Strawberries, banana, almond drain, and a sprinkle of nectar.

10. Outlandish Elude:

Mango, pineapple, coconut water, and a sprinkle of lime.

5 Fruit-Infused Water Formulas for Hydration:

1. Strawberry and Mint Refresher
2. Lemon and Lime Zinger
3. Cucumber and Grapefruit Cooler
4. Orange and Ginger Energizer
5. Berry Rapture (blend of blueberries, raspberries, and blackberries)

3 Fruit-Based Dessert Formulas for a Sweet Treat:

1. Barbecued Pineapple with Coconut Ice Cream
2. Strawberry Banana Decent Cream (made with solidified bananas and strawberries)
3. Mango Sorbet with a sprinkle of lime

These fruit blends are not as it were scrumptious but too pressed with supplements, vitamins, and cancer prevention agents to keep you energized and hydrated all through the day! So go ahead, get inventive, and enjoy these delicious treats! Your taste buds and body will really appreciate you!

Conclusion: Embracing a Fruitful Life!

Wow, what a ride! We've investigated the dynamic world of fruits, revealing their privileged insights, and finding the extraordinary benefits they bring to our lives. From boosting our wellbeing and vitality to rousing inventiveness and delight, natural products are genuinely a blessing from nature!

Outline of Key Focuses:

- Fruits are filled with supplements, vitamins, and cancer prevention agents that supercharge our bodies and minds.
- Joining an assortment of fruits into our day by day and eating less can have a critical effect on our by and large prosperity.
- Fruit blends and smoothies are a tasty and helpful way to appreciate the benefits of fruits In our life.
- Fruit-infused water and sweets offer a reviving and sweet way to remain hydrated and fulfilled.
- Grasping a productive living can bring us closer to nature, rouse inventiveness, and cultivate a sense of community.

Support to Grasp a Productive Living:

As we conclude this travel, keep in mind that each fruit encompasses a story to tell and an advantage to share. By grasping a fruity living, you're not as it were feeding your body but moreover developing a more profound association with nature and the world around you. So go ahead, investigate the dynamic world of fruits, and find the unimaginable benefits they bring to your life!

Appreciation

A gigantic thank you to each and each one of you who has joined me on this productive experience! Your excitement and adore for natural products have made this travel a supreme charm. In case you've delighted in this book, it would be ideal if you take a minute to take off an audit and share your favorite fruit minutes with others. Your reviews will mean the world to me, and I can't wait to hear approximately your fruitful encounters!

Keep in mind, a fruity life may be a cheerful life! Keep sparkling, and let the fruitiness rouse you each day!

Acknowledgments: A Fruitful Thank You!

Composing this book has been an extraordinary experience, and I'm so thankful to have had the back of a few astounding people along the way. Here's a huge, delicious thank you to:

-       My editors, who made a difference me prune my thoughts and shape them into something excellent
-       My technicians, who brought the book to life with their dynamic outlines and format

-       My individual natural product devotees,
who shared their energy and skill with me
-       My family and companions, who energized
me to keep going, indeed when the composing got
extreme
-       And of course, the fruits themselves, for
being so scrumptiously rousing!

Much obliged to each and each one of you, this
book is presently in your hands, and I trust it brings
a burst of enhance and delight to your life!

NOTE

NOTE

NOTE

NOTE